Eugene's Gift

Nerelle Poroch

Eugene's Gift

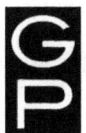

Eugene's Gift
ISBN 978 1 74027 122 6
Copyright © Nerelle Poroch 2019

First published 2001
Reprinted 2020

Ginninderra Press
PO Box 3461 Port Adelaide 5015
www.ginninderrapress.com.au

This book is dedicated to the recipients of the gift.

Introduction

This is the story of Eugene's gift to those he knew. Those who experienced his willingness to change his outlook on life in a bid to continue living were inspired by his gift of sharing a wonderful 'moment' in life with him. Others only saw his life cut short at forty-six by stomach cancer; a cancer presumed to be reserved only for the elderly.

During surgery to remove his stomach, the doctor had found that Eugene's cancer was inoperable because of the extensive spread into other areas and its effect on vital blood vessels near it. He had a level four cancer with little hope of recovery. Following the operation, Eugene started to attend cancer self help group sessions at the ACT Cancer Society in Canberra for relaxation, meditation and group support. He was the only male in a group of, on average, six to ten women.

From the group he learned of the various alternative and traditional medical help the other cancer sufferers had followed. He was told about their addiction to meditation and its healing powers.

He also learned about the dietary beliefs of the fellow-sufferers and the alternative therapy they had sought from people like Ian Gawler and Gerry Manion, who conduct live-in cancer seminars for sufferers and their carers. These seminars are essentially about putting mind, spirit and body in balance and creating a positive environment to get well.

Another significant source of help was Jen Luddington, a naturopath based in Canberra who had assisted other cancer patients in balancing mind, spirit and body.

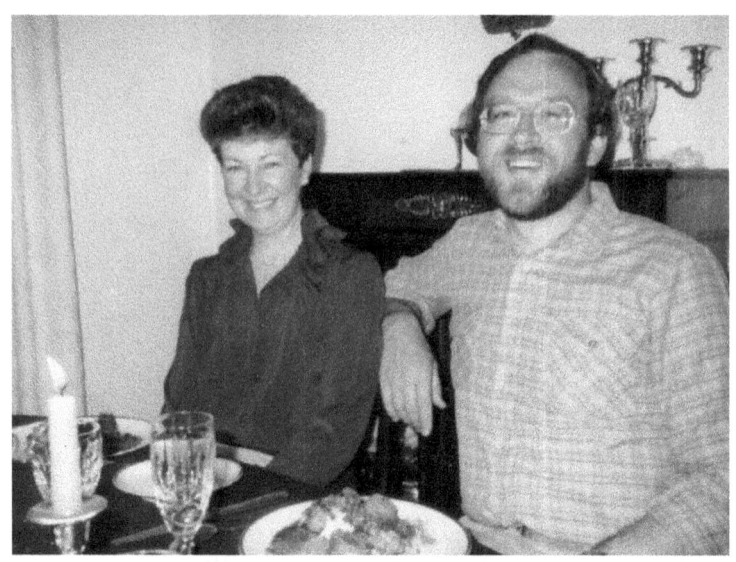

Nerelle and Eugene, March 1988

The spirit evident in the cancer support group room at the ACT Cancer Society, where sufferers support each other, is very uplifting. It was a privileged and a powerful place to be present as Eugene's wife and carer, supporting another on such a journey. The individual's background is irrelevant in this situation. The strength that each one gives the other is all that counts.

In the days and months to come, Eugene was to become an inspiration to others in the group in bearing his cancer with increasing dignity the more it progressed. Through contact with other cancer sufferers, he allowed himself exposure to further information and philosophies, which included meditation, the benefits of betacarotene (carrot juice), special diets, vitamins, chemotherapy, naturopathy, shark's cartilage powder and faith in God.

From being incapable of making changes to improve his working life over the previous nineteen years, Eugene embraced his six-month journey through cancer with an open mind and with unlimited energy and confidence.

Preface

'Alas for those who never sing, but die with all their music in them.' – Oliver Wendell Holmes

The legacy Eugene has left us all is in how he answered the challenge of cancer. His was not a fight against something as mysteriously elusive as cancer. That was the job of his immune system. His was a more positive response that had him fight for life itself as the prime objective. It is the difference between healing – making whole – and curing.

> 'The real miracle happens when the patient sees physical recovery as merely an ancillary, and regards the gift of living life fully as the primary and essential benefit.' – Russell Lockhart

Cancer is an ultimatum for profound change.

'We must never forget that we may find meaning in life even when confronted with a hopeless situation. When facing a fate that cannot be changed, when we are no longer able to change a situation, we are challenged to change ourselves.' – Viktor Frankl

When we find someone meeting the challenge of change, such change, to find meaning and purpose in their life, as Eugene so courageously did, we are in awe and admiration.

In the Introduction, Dr Poroch tells us that Eugene, after much suffering, lost his life. It is a perfect example of the paradox we read about in Matthew 10:39 when Jesus said, 'Whoever loses his life will find it.'

We are indebted to Nerelle for this intimate story that will provide inspiration for all who read it thoughtfully. Her modesty in minimising her role cannot conceal its vital importance. This is a love story, and so a story of two people, whose love for one another united them in such a way that their stories are one.

Our work with cancer patients led us to the awareness of the significance of being and belonging – and of being where you belong. How appropriate that Nerelle helped Eugene find his way to be at home in this life, and to remain there till eventually he really did find his way home. In this way they became a blessing to each other.

Gerard Manion
Home Hospice Inc., Bundeena

Carl Simonton, MD in the treatment of cancer, believes that illness is a negative feedback system. It is telling us what we need to stop doing. He considers that looking at illness in this way has great value. It might be telling us that we need to modify our work habits, to rest or to question what we are doing. It helps us stop doing things that are counterproductive. It helps us align ourselves. More importantly, it forces us to reach out for help, bringing more love to us. Illness can help us connect a deeper, more loving more cooperative way with people around us, rather than isolate ourselves.

This is what happened during Eugene's journey. He grew to be what Dr Bernie Siegel has termed 'the exceptional cancer patient', in that he changed many aspects of his life and asked questions and took risks in the process of improving the quality of his life. The exceptional cancer patient is totally willing to participate, to be assertive and communicative. This was evidenced in Eugene's approach in communicating with the medical profession, where he would prepare lists of questions in order to understand fully his condition. He also looked at the total picture of his life. He was not afraid to examine or share his feelings and not afraid to change. He was flexible enough to shed the old patterns of living associated with the cancer-producing physiology (feeling negative, impatient and stressed) and to become psychologically whole. Dr Siegel considers that despair suppresses people's immune systems. He considers that when you teach people to survive through living, loving and laughing you are working through the immune system.

Eugene reached out for help in all of these areas. In approaching faith in God, he felt he was not worthy to attend the local church's healing service because, if it had not been for his illness, he would not have sought this type of help. He also could not relate to a strong belief in God's help. However, on attending his first healing service, Eugene was overwhelmed at the generosity of the minister and his parishioners, who laid hands on him and prayed for his healing. In a prayer of reply, Eugene stated that he felt a fraud in coming to the service because he needed help and he would not have otherwise considered attending. The parishioners assured him that he should receive gladly their prayers and best wishes.

He had taken a risk on unfamiliar ground with strangers praying for him and needing to communicate his gratitude in response to their generosity. He was reminded of the philosophy of Susan Jeffers' book *Feel the Fear and Do It Anyway*. He used the spirit of this title when he plunged in to make his prayer of thanks to God when it was his turn. After the service, he went up to each person and thanked them individually for their generosity. Their very generous and giving nature evoked a spontaneous growth in Eugene's ability to show his gratitude for their charity in allowing him to be the centre of attention in asking God's help in his healing.

In the days to come, Eugene was to contemplate the writings of many thinkers, including the Reverend Jim Glennon, who started the healing services in Sydney's City Anglican Cathedral, whose prayer appealed to him:

> Blessed Lord, who prayed all night when the need was great, help me to pray all day for my great need and give me of your wisdom that I will pray aright. I believe that as my prayer of faith continues, you are casting my mountain into the sea, spadeful by spadeful. I have faith to affirm that in the best and truest sense your will is being done on earth as it is in heaven and that, in this difficulty, I and mine are being changed into your likeness more and more. Lord Jesus, my hand is in yours; I will not let you go unless you bless me.

He also considered Kathryn Kuhlman's writing on faith:

> Faith is a gift of God or a fruit of the Spirit, and whether it be gift

or fruit, the source and the origin of faith remain the same. It comes from God and is a gift of God. If faith is powerless, it is not faith. You cannot have faith without results any more than you can have motion without movement. The thing we sometimes call faith, is only trust, but although we trust in the Lord, it is faith which has action and power.

And Ram Dass, a spiritual teacher in meditation in the United States, talks about climbing one's mountain during a lifetime; he considers that a few reach the top of the mountain to experience the mystic experience every great climber has known. He also sees the path of the mountain reflected in Christ's forty days in the desert in gaining enlightenment:

Who returns from the top of the mountain comes back quietness itself, is compassion and wisdom, is the truth of the ages. He or she becomes a light for others on the way, a statement of the freedom that comes from having touched the top of the mountain.

Ram Dass also cites Rene Daumal's thoughts:

You cannot stay on the summit forever; you have to come down again... So why bother in the first place? Just this: what is above knows what is below, but what is below does not know what is above. One climbs, one sees. One descends, one sees no longer but one has seen. There is an art to conducting oneself in the lower regions by the memory of what one saw higher up. When one can no longer see, one can at least still know.

Eugene's journey can be likened to Ram Dass's view that up to the very end of the climb up the mountain of liberation the most subtle suffering still remains, for there is still an individual who identifies with his or her own separateness. There is still clinging. There is still a final bond to break. At the moment of scaling the highest peak, the climber must let go of everything, even self-consciousness, in order to become the perfect instrument of the climb. In the ultimate moments of the climb, he or she transcends even the identity of the climber. Christ said one must truly die and be born again.

The absence of identity with personal ego, which Eugene was to learn about, means that the being is free, is pure compassion, pure love, pure awareness. For such a being, everything is in the moment. There is a richness in which past, present and future all coexist.

Eugene was to become enlightened, realised, free and a child of God.

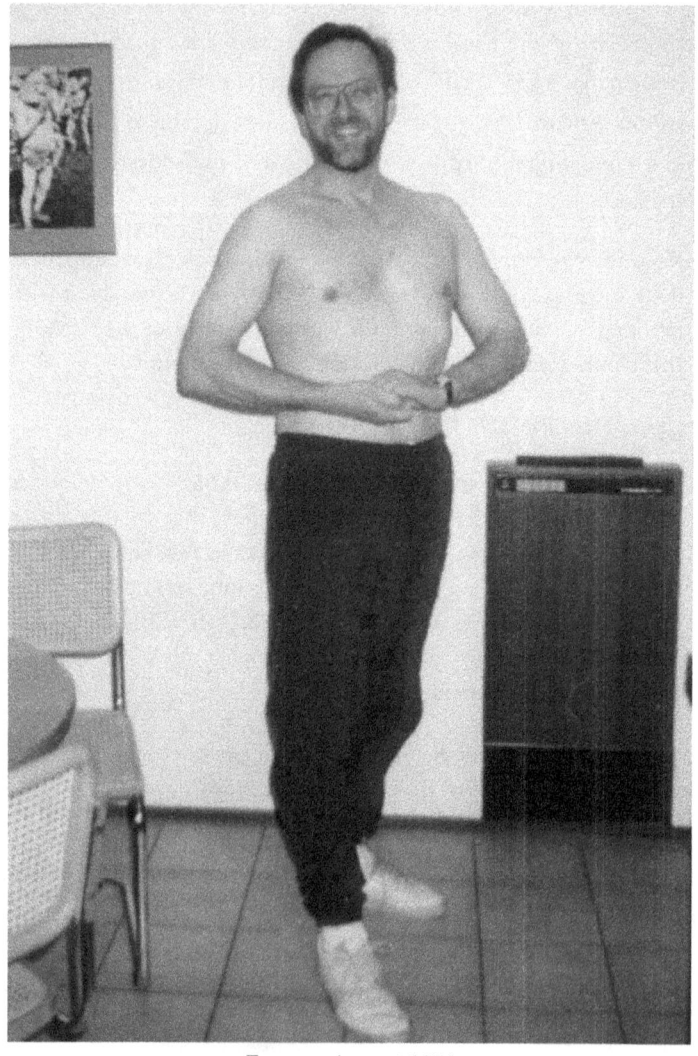

Eugene, August 1994

Eugene's first step on this journey was to experience Gerry Manion's cancer care program at Bundeena in NSW. This was a period of five days with morning and afternoon sessions with Gerry of intensive counselling for both patient and carer. The program was to equip Eugene for the long and complex journey ahead and nothing could have been more appropriately based in changing his whole outlook.

In the daily sessions, Gerry worked with Eugene on examining the life stresses that led up to his illness. Eugene learned to meditate to visualise positive messages such as the strong T cells eating the weak cancer cells. He also learned deep relaxation and the importance of acknowledging breathing – the outward sign of the inner spirit – and of gentle exercise such as walking.

He was also taught about the immune system, how it works and how he could influence it by positive thinking. Finding freedom from those things that had inhibited his life in the past was explored in depth and through practical exercises, so that he was able to explore options and to clarify his real needs. As an example, he learned how to release emotions. He was introduced to ways of freeing the inner child and to the value of the belly laugh and reassessing the beliefs which lead to behaviour. This reassessment leads to new ways of being, relating and creating and to an ability to adopt new attitudes in line with clearer thinking. He was then led into the realm of setting goals out of the belief and purpose in life.

Gerry's priority is happiness. He considers that the participant in his cancer care program is the exceptional patient who wants to learn new ways of living, to become free to be fully oneself without fear to sing one's own individual song at the physical, mental and spiritual level. He considers that a life-threatening illness can present this opportunity and sees cancer as an ultimatum for profound change. The primary aim of the participants in the program is to learn to respond daily with the most satisfying, purposeful, joyful living – free to be themselves, growing daily towards becoming the person they have the potential to be. Thus, they provide their immune systems with the optimum atmosphere in which to function. In also helping the carer with the stress of caring for a loved one, Gerry opens up the opportunity for more meaningful communication and openness, an enhanced relationship, a time for loving and caring – a time for living.

During the week with Gerry, Eugene was asked to use his imagination to find out who was the real and unique Eugene. He was asked to write out a wish list of 'freedom from' and 'freedom to do' certain things and 'twenty ways to play'. Eugene found difficulty in using his imagination to prepare these lists. He was unable to respond to music by dancing, as he was extremely self-conscious. Following Simonton's philosophy, Gerry told Eugene that using our imagination is one of the most effective ways to build belief. The more we imagine, the more we create a climate for a whole new view. The more we accept this new view, the more we allow understanding to begin as we practise it. That is what permits us to overcome illness.

In his wish to get everything right, Eugene had many fears that he was not doing enough and that his meditation method was incorrect. He was also concerned that he was not convinced about following the many strict diets prescribed for cancer sufferers in the literature he had been reading. Gerry's advice was that he should not force meditation – it happens. His views on diet were to eat everything in moderation and not to adopt radical diets.

Gerry introduced Eugene to his concepts of using the will to love. He considers that love is employing the will to love – that is, choosing to love oneself; getting rid of resentments; finding one's spirituality; experiencing the value of the hug, signifying belonging; reverting to childhood and re-examining the early beliefs which lead to what we become and have a bearing on our behaviour. Consequently, he emphasised the importance of having fun; of loving oneself in order to love others; and the need to reach one's potential through the imagination. He emphasised that problems are caused by negative imagination: we need to use assertiveness in creating positive imagination. Eugene's favourite phrase for many years had been 'it's hopeless', which had summarised much of his recent attitude towards life.

Through Gerry's program, Eugene was given the opportunity to assess the constraints which he had placed on his life and the need to be free from self-imposed constraints. For Eugene, these were dependence on other people; fear of ridicule, fear of failure, fear of attempting new things or jobs; being boring, directionless, having low self-esteem, being criticised; the drudgery of everyday life, loneliness, not having any definite purpose; and the fear of approaching people for help and friendship.

Through Gerry's program, Eugene realised that he had to change his whole way of thinking about his life, that he had to find himself through the principles of self, which are to be, to belong and to steer a course. He needed to use maturity, which is awareness, acceptance and confidence (obtained through imagination), and find balance, which is the control of emotions and the will to love. He needed to learn that mental health is both vigour and peace; that cancer is the problem; and that he needed to focus on the solution – that is, the enjoyment of life. Gerry told him that no one had died of laughter! He stressed that, when we can't change the situation, we are then challenged to change ourselves and this was the essence of what Eugene was to work on.

Eugene's expectations of Gerry's program were that, on completing the program, everything would be clear-cut, including the way to meditate. However, he learnt that there is no formula. It is all to be found within one's self. Eugene needed to work on what he had learnt. He had to change. Eugene was the problem but he was also the solution.

During the week with Gerry, he also attended the Wednesday night Healing Service at the Sydney City Anglican Cathedral, where he experienced the generosity of strangers in praying for him. The poignancy of his situation was highlighted by the service. In a ritual for the sick, the minister also anointed him. Eugene had wanted very much to attend this service and to stay on and chat afterwards, and he spoke to people during the tea and cakes that followed the service, which was very much out of character.

Eugene returned to Canberra wondering how he was to employ all of Gerry's advice and so become a balanced person. He had learned to visualise making the T cells (the white cells) eat up the cancer cells through positive thinking and visualisation during meditation. But how was he to find himself, be at peace, not be stressed and impatient, and find spirituality? The day he left the house on the cliff at Bundeena was the first time he accomplished packing and cleaning up without stress and impatience. The growth had begun.

Gerry's initial legacy on Eugene's homecoming was his appreciation of the value of the gift of the hug. It gave strength and love and support and a sense of belonging.

From this time onwards, we were to experience the cocoon of love extended by eight close friends. A loving and support ive time of regularly dining together and sharing happy times followed. This provided the fun times recommended by Gerry, which were supplemented by humorous movies and books, and enjoying favourite places. Three of Eugene's work colleagues were also to give a solid wall of support throughout his illness. His mother, two brothers, sister and nephew visited from Perth and provided family love and support.

The medical advice suggested that Eugene would be wise to embark on a radical course of chemotherapy, which, in view of his relative youth, his system could sustain. At the same time, Eugene had taken Gerry's advice and considered what his goals were in the future. They were to visit his family in Perth and to visit Egypt, Italy and Israel. However, he was advised that it would be prudent to embark on the chemotherapy treatment without delay. After three sessions, he would be reassessed to see if his stomach tumour had reduced.

For his first session, Eugene spent three days in hospital hooked up to the chemotherapy, a hydration drip and a blood transfusion. He had listened to Gerry's guided imagery tapes while the treatment progressed and tried to imagine the chemotherapy killing off the cancerous cells. He returned home feeling rather depressed, with fevers and sweating which were ever present throughout his illness. He felt very weak and unable to come to grips with the depression following all that he had experienced in hospital. For each procedure, there had been a deal of trouble finding his veins that had worried him. He had not expected to feel so let down after the first treatment of chemotherapy, which he viewed as a last resort, and had resolved that this treatment, together with his positive thinking, would enable him to beat the cancer. In spite of these resolves and attitudes, he worried that having the chemotherapy had resulted in his having a negative outlook. He had been generally overwhelmed by all the treatment and had found that its effects made it difficult for him to take in Gerry's tapes. His ability to concentrate on the treatment destroying the cancer cells was also diminished through the impulse to sleep during treatment.

After recording all the events of his chemotherapy session and its aftermath, he found that the act of writing about these recent experiences helped and he resolved to return to his routine of meditation. It was also very difficult for Eugene to forget about the possible side-effects of the treatment which his oncologist had highlighted, as he was feeling extremely weak. Contact with the community nurses and the Palliative Care Nursing Service, which was later to become paramount in his life, was also initiated after his first chemotherapy treatment.

The Cancer Society information had led him to Jen Luddington, a naturopath who uses touch for healing, kinesiology and Bowen techniques. His first session with Jen was two days after he returned home from hospital. Jen was to assist Eugene in putting Gerry's philosophy into practice. She advised him to get rid of his seriousness; to consciously make the opportunity of having fun; to write about relationships – specific people, the resentments in his life, his surroundings, his past and present worries and to get in touch with his spiritual self. She emphasised the need to know who he was and to experience feelings as she considered he was unable to do this. He found it very difficult to describe himself for Jen. After much thought, he recorded his characteristics:

kind	dependable
appreciate and enjoy plays, movies, music	reliable
steady	friendly
listen to people	sensitive

love books	decent
competent	sense of humour

Eugene was a big-boned well covered man of six-foot – somewhat like a Russian bear. To be with Eugene was immensely enjoyable because of his sense of humour. He was also a great worrier about everything from missing trains to his own health. He would comment with gusto about news items in the media, and around the house would emit loud, humorous shouts. Notwithstanding his reluctance to attend social occasions, after a few drinks he would do outrageous things such as dancing on the dinner table at a restaurant or seating himself in the Governor General's Rolls Royce at an official ceremony.

His uniqueness was his honesty and forthrightness. He maintained a great interest in reading about politics, sport, history, biographies and current affairs. He was continually frustrated by the fact that people in general indulge in small talk that he was unable to conduct. He constantly felt the need to discuss and talk about the topics he was reading. Only one friend, Barry, had debated such topics with him over a twenty-year period. During their discussions, Eugene forcefully took the opposite viewpoint.

It was usual for Eugene during a car journey of four hours to talk non-stop about these favourite topics. He was a wonderful communicator in being able to impart the information he obtained from reading, although he was always bemoaning the fact that he had read so many books but forgot their contents on putting them down. He constantly had a book in his hand and devoured the newspapers each day. He could be dogmatic in his views and was amused and bewildered, when airing his views around the dinner table, that no one would be listening.

Eugene cared that any activity, whether work or playing cards, was carried out correctly. He was the leader and the organiser in recording the scores of card games, in planning and enjoying holidays and in looking after financial matters. He would carry out a job in the garden while counting the number of barrow loads and the time it took to fill each load. He loved recording sporting statistics and maintained a project for over twenty years where he recorded Australian Rules, cricket and federal election results in a variety of ways.

After the first session with Jen, he recorded in his diary that he felt more positive than during the days following the first chemotherapy session. He was in this frame of mind when his brother Alex arrived from Perth the following day with his young son Tom. Eugene was very weak during the first part of their visit and hardly able to conduct a conversation. Nevertheless, his observance of Gerry's and Jen's advice was evident during the visit when he examined his usual reaction of impatience and worry about an eight-year-old's exuberance in terms of damaging items in the house. He recorded in his diary, 'Tom is a worry. I should just let go. I am too staid. No wonder I need to lighten up.' He sympathised with his brother's frustration in his own particular work situation and comments, 'We all have some fears regarding jobs and doing them.'

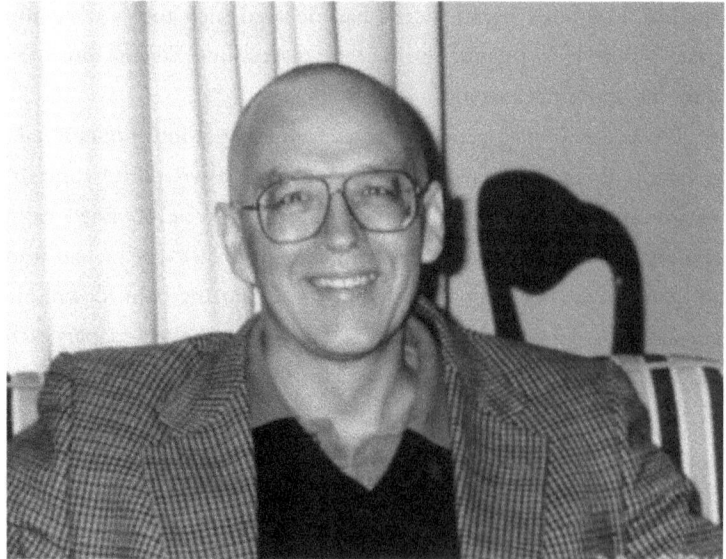

Eugene, October 1994

From now on, Eugene was to record his daily eating habits, the people he spoke to, his activities, his medical side-effects, his sleep patterns and his feelings. Some of his comments on relationships include:

> Siblings: Very good relationships.
>
> Friends: Have few close friends. In recent years perhaps not as much involvement as should. Lack of confidence in dealing with people.
>
> Other friends and acquaintances: I get on well with people but normally leave it up to them to contact me rather than me doing the contacting. This is in part due to being part of a couple and leaving up to my wife to do most of the contact.
>
> Work: Generally good – I would say most people would say I'm easy to work with. Only one unpleasant relationship.

On past resentments of various duration, he writes of resentment towards:

> Some fellow workers because of their attitude to work.
>
> Having the feeling that I've been left with the job.
>
> My supervisors for lack of support.
>
> One particular worker for trying to undermine me (in my view).
>
> When young towards parents, who expected too much of me because I was the eldest child.
>
> A close friend in Canberra when he developed a relationship and other interests which appeared then to exclude me.

The following comment after listing these resentments indicates Eugene's success in putting his life into perspective:

I believe I've got rid of most if not all of them (the resentments) – hard to say. I know much of it does not matter at all.

He was able to record the things, apart from friends, family and work colleagues, that indicated he was not alone as:

The garden – which I really enjoy.
Books – my library gives me great pleasure.
Doing the washing.
Where I live.
Birds in the trees.

During this time of recovery from the chemotherapy, Eugene sat in the garden, enjoying his brother's company. Taking Jen's advice seriously, he made a considerable effort to take the initiative in communicating and meeting various friends – something he was not in the habit of doing previously. He also made a point of watching humorous movies and taking walks with his brother and nephew. He had always enjoyed the easy and light-hearted company of his two brothers and sister whenever they met. This easy style of family interaction now came to the fore. Friends also locked into the habit of regularly calling and enjoying socialising over lunch and dinner. Eugene enjoyed these times immensely.

As a member of the cancer support group, he gained enormous benefit and growth from the other members' ability to share and communicate their feelings in a loving and accepting way. The only male in the group, he was privileged to be part of women's ability to share their experience of cancer frankly and to give steadfast support. In reaching out to others, he found that the cancer support group gave him immeasurable help in being able to share his experiences with others in the same circumstances. For instance, he was able to obtain help in role-modelling after hearing Marjory's story of how she overcame her cancer through adopting a positive attitude in the face of death.

Jen had commented that his problem was that he had excluded the growth of the spiritual dimension of his person. She said that all parts must be in balance and somewhere in the past this aspect had not been allowed to develop. Similarly with his emotional self. She observed that he was a logical person and had developed this aspect only. On these issues he records in his diary, 'Must work on the other sides if I'm to help in a cure and feeling whole.'

Jen had suggested he read spiritual texts (the Bible or any of the religious works); visit consecrated ground (such as churches); listen to music such as Gregorian chants; relate to nature – all food for the spiritual self. Eugene put this into practice by sitting quietly in churches, listening to music, reading the Bible and attending the healing ministry at a local church. The healing sessions were a great source of strength in his growing belief that it was worth giving faith in God a go. All of these measures resulted in his increased feeling of confidence. He also rang various friends to reciprocate their concern, which was totally out of character in terms of his attitude in the past. By being able to achieve a balance in his life and within the strong cocoon of friends' and family's love, he was able to minimise the gravity of his illness until the approach of each chemotherapy session, which by the time they were due also heralded a significant reduction in his stamina.

During the last two chemotherapy sessions, Eugene gained one week of being well in every three, when he felt strong and able to enjoy good quality of life. During this period, he worked on keeping a balance in his life by putting joy into it. This was done during intense social activity with the friends and family. His brother John and his sister Tanya visited from Perth, and his mother commuted between Perth and Canberra during Eugene's illness. There was constant contact on the phone with friends, dinners at restaurants and at friends' homes, constant outings to movies and other places which had given enjoyment in the past and which continued to provide enjoyment in Eugene's wavering state of health during the chemotherapy. He was also aware and concerned about its possible help versus its potential to cause damage to healthy organs.

He continued to see Jen Luddington and embarked on meditation sessions with Sri Chinmoy as well as the cancer support group. He records in his diary at this time that he was feeling good generally. He was also able to give an upbeat description of his own situation at the cancer

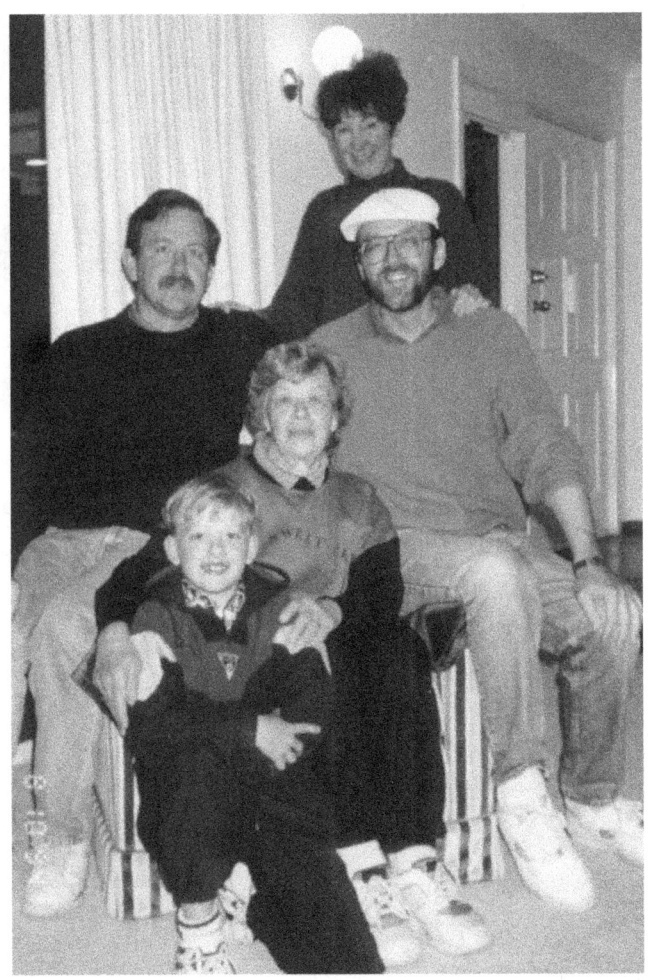

Eugene, with Alex, Tom and his mother Anna, October 1994

support group when the group was sharing personal feelings. He became an inspiration to other members of the group due to his strong optimism and strength of belief when he was obviously being intensely affected by the chemotherapy in weight loss (now reduced to seventy-four kilograms from ninety), loss of hair and loss of stamina – he was unable to regain his appetite and strength for any long period of time.

Eugene's demeanour and appearance was changing markedly as he

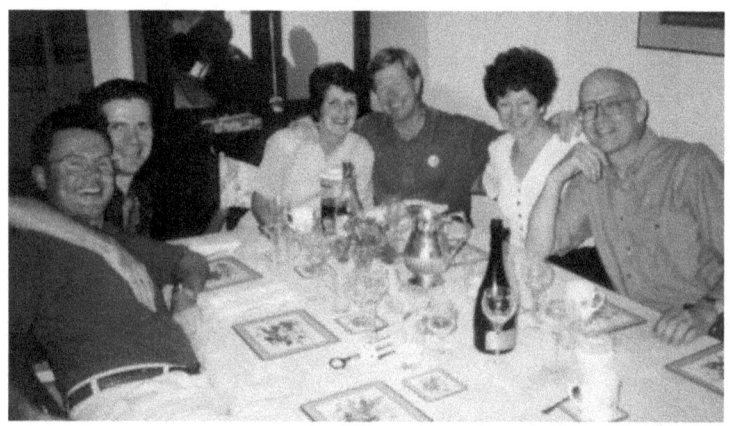

Eugene with friends Barry, Steve, Pam and Cliff, November 1994

had been a heavy-handed, clumsy person whose gait was unpredictable, and often walked in other people's space. Now he was becoming very regal. His friends in the cancer support group described his demeanour as very dignified. A work colleague did not recognise him at this time due to these changes. Once he adjusted to having a shaven head, he exposed it with dignity and even grew to like the way he looked. The inner glow of finding himself was becoming obvious in his face. He was able to feel for friends' happy and sad life experiences.

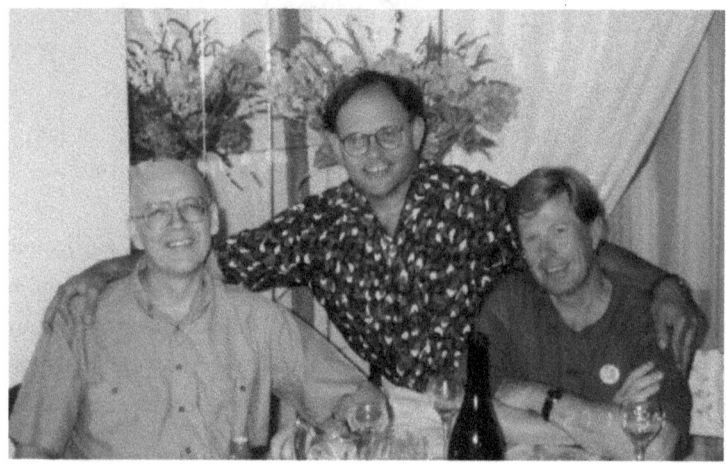

Eugene with friends Barry, Steve, Pam and Cliff, November 1994

All of his friends were very comfortable in being with Eugene and in the way he was handling his illness. His attitude to the cancer was such that no one felt that there was any need to treat him differently from the way they had in the past.

He enjoyed light-hearted chat and laughter when George, a friend, photographed him in an old moth-eaten wig, which he tried on after he had his head shaved.

Mindful of Gerry's advice about setting goals for himself, Eugene decided at this time that the most important thing to do after visiting his family in Perth was to journey to Egypt, Italy and Israel. Planning for this trip provided the feeling that it would happen, and he was able to conclude that in six months he would embark on the trip and he would be 'well and truly on top of the cancer by then'. At the very least, he had high hopes of gaining at least six months of good health following the chemotherapy treatment.

When Gerry Manion visited his cancer support group, he did not recognise Eugene at first due to his weight and hair loss. Eugene was overjoyed at seeing Gerry again and showed his feelings without the usual restraint he had maintained in his past life. Eugene had also developed a certain aura of calm and happiness by this time, to the extent that it was as if those close to him were caught up in a deep breath of life, love, happiness and peace of mind.

Eugene was feeling well, if a little weak, and eating normally at the time of a subsequent visit to Sydney to consult a medical practitioner about the benefit of treatment overseas and shark's cartilage treatment. He experienced discomfort in the stomach on the journey home. The next day, Eugene had to undergo a CT scan and an X-ray to determine whether the three sessions of chemotherapy had been in any way successful. During the tests, he became very ill, with intense pain in the abdomen. Further tests showed a partial blockage of the bowel. Heavy night sweats accompanied the intense pain. He needed to be admitted to hospital but there was a lack of beds. He was caught in bureaucracy, which determined he could only be admitted in an emergency which was life-threatening. By the time he attended his appointment with the oncologist for the results of the CT scan, his stomach had started to extend from the tumour.

It was a terrible blow when the medical tests and subsequent examination showed that the tumour had not decreased at all and had indeed grown. He was annoyed that his regular doctor, whom he trusted, had asked the registrar to break the news. The reason was that the registrar would be able to give more time, and answer all the questions following the news. After an hour's consultation, Eugene sat in the waiting area and shed tears at the loss of his strong hopes for an extended life.

In essence, the registrar's advice was that, in spite of the chemotherapy treatment, the tumour had grown and other cancerous nodules were evident. Morphine was prescribed for the pain, with the hope that the bowel would become less constricted with time. Eugene's poor physical condition would not allow any consideration of an operation to rectify the blockage. A lesser dosage of chemotherapy was prescribed each week, and this treatment gave only a fifteen per cent chance of making any improvement. Nevertheless, this was a small lifeline as well as a sign of not giving up hope at this low stage. The hospital dietician gave advice about a liquid diet that Eugene needed now, as he was not able to take solids.

How does a person accept such news after having such high hopes for improvement which would extend life? Eugene became unsure of future plans regarding other possible treatment, his proposed holiday overseas and visit to Perth. He had negative dreams about his cancer, which again motivated him to extend his exploration of areas of assistance and self-help in overcoming the cancer. He booked a live-in cancer seminar with Ian Gawler in Melbourne in the following months. He arranged to obtain a quantity of shark's cartilage without delay from a Queensland supplier.

In the following days and weeks, the palliative care nurses provided education on how to maintain the adequate dosage of morphine to keep ahead of Eugene's increasing pain, as well as dietary arrangements in the face of his decreasing ability to digest food. Each palliative care nurse brought her own individual help and special skills in comforting mind, spirit and body. They brought items that would make Eugene more comfortable. Above all, they understood that cancer bestows on its bearers and carers a very privileged time for those who grasp the opportunity of the unique experience which it offers in all of its associated tragedy.

During the next two months, Eugene's world progressively became smaller in that he was restricted to sitting in the garden, then the lounge room and finally to the bedroom. He also reached the stage where he needed a wheelchair at the hospital door on the occasion of each chemotherapy visit and after a few sessions was unable to visit the hospital to continue the chemotherapy treatment. The doctor at this time decided that it was taking up strength that he needed and it was discontinued. From a solid six-foot, ninety-kilogram man, he was reduced to a very frail and weakened state. It became necessary for friends not to visit for a time while he was adapting to increasing pain and attaining adequate morphine pain management.

The minister from the healing ministry now started calling to the house with Communion on Sundays. Eugene looked forward to these visits. His prayers to his God during these visits were an inspiration. They revealed how far he had travelled from the day when Jen introduced him to getting in touch with his spirituality and he replied that he had no conception of what she meant or wanted him to achieve – he was strictly into the tangible and logical at that time.

On Eugene's last visit to Jen Luddington, she said that she could sense his new self and commented on how he had changed. He had grown into a much softer and caring person who was able to freely give and receive love. Whilst Eugene was still fighting for his life, he had also found inner peace and happiness. He had fused together all the learning he had taken in since his time with Gerry and was reaching his point of fulfilment.

The correct pain management through morphine was vital to enable him to enjoy friends' visits and their love and support, which was a necessary part of this stage of his illness. His physical condition was rapidly changing and he was becoming thinner and weaker. Each visit the friends made was short and they were shocked by his rapid deterioration. During a work colleague's visit, he tapped Eugene on the arm as he was telling him a story. Eugene was so weak that he was compelled to tell his friend that he was hurting him.

George and Cliff offered practical help in renovating his pyjamas to accommodate the growing tumour in his stomach. Thinking back a year, it was impossible to imagine that a sewing production line for Eugene would be necessary – unpicking stitches, sewing Velcro and rethreading the cord. It was very frustrating for friends to know that there was little else they could do for Eugene. They marvelled that he looked so clean and fetching amidst the ravages of the disease and at his wonderful attitude of mind when talking about the happy times together and insisting, 'We'll do it again!' His newfound spirituality was also obvious in the last visits which the friends enjoyed with him in his peacefulness and calmness and loving attitude towards them.

This softer, gentler way of living had become obvious in the early days of his decrease in health, when he would watch humorous movies until late at night and sit in the garden during the day. As the pain intensified, he was confined to the lounge room and later, when he became weaker, the bedroom chair. He had asked the doctor how long he had to live, but not to pinpoint any time (that is, in his words, 'not to point the bone'). He had read in the cancer literature that patients tend to lock in on such a timeframe. When the doctor mentioned that he was not looking at a year, Eugene visualised that he had many months of life ahead of him, when in fact his death was only a month away.

Elizabeth Kubler-Ross has found through her work with the dying that, for people who are in harmony with their own physical, emotional, intellectual and spiritual quadrants, death can be a graduation. They die when they have learned their lessons – after they have taught and learned what they need to teach and learn. This was the way with Eugene.

However, whilst learning the lessons and facing the inevitable, it can still be difficult to know how far one can debate with another about the finality of a life which is ending. This was particularly so with Eugene, as he had such an intense resolve to beat the disease. To speak about the alternative to life seemed to go against what his only focus was about. However, his fight for life also did not allow him to stop the fight when he possibly needed to. This became obvious when one night he dreamed that his cancer was cured and that everything was going to be all right. He described it as a wonderful, happy dream but was worried that the ending was not correct, as he had dreamed that he would be cured and he knew that this was not going to happen. He could not bear to speak in terms that he would not have to suffer much longer and soon the pain would be over. His logical mind was so attuned to keeping alive to an unspecified point in the future that he could not bear to think that his time was fast approaching.

Eugene was finding it difficult now to speak on the phone with friends and relatives. At this time, he asked me how his cancer had affected me apart from the worry and the concern of looking after him. I told him that the gift he had bestowed on me in his illness was the search for spirituality and the privilege of caring wholly for his well-being. I had also learned to receive gladly the support and love of friends and to recognise a positive attitude, as opposed to the negativity of those who are unable to live balanced lives and to provide support to others. I told him that he allowed me to share a very privileged time with him which I would never experience again in my lifetime.

Eugene was admitted to hospital in need of a blood transfusion, as his haemoglobin was very low. It took from ten p.m. until four a.m. the following morning for him to be settled in the cancer ward after going through the outpatients department. I felt very concerned and protective of his need for one-to-one care and continued to shower him and to give him morphine brought from home when the nurses were late in administering the dose. These were very difficult days, when I had to battle the hospital system for an available hospital bed for Eugene's urgent needs.

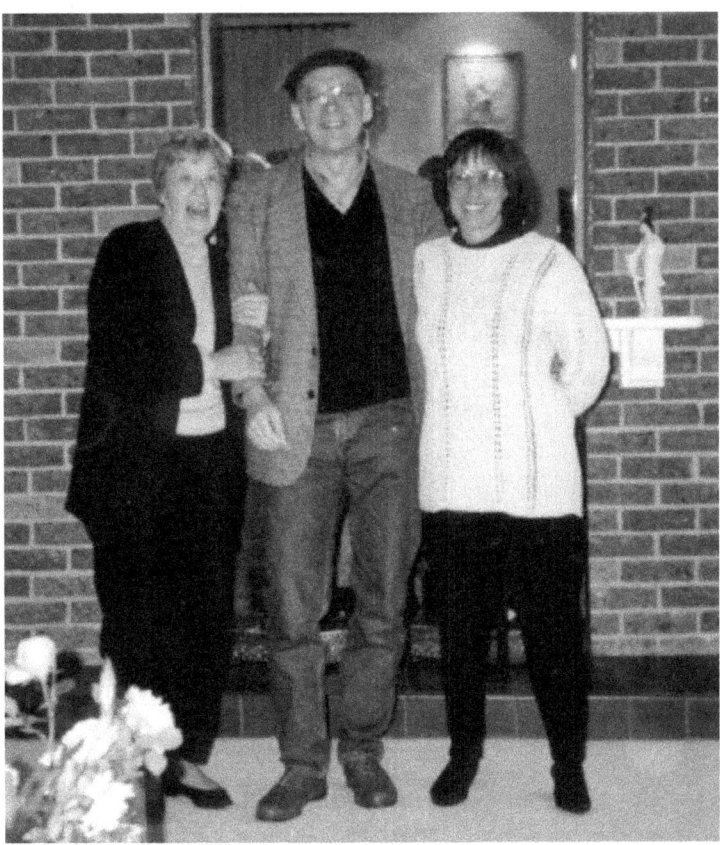

Eugene with Anna and Tanya, October 1994

While in hospital, Eugene wanted his oncologist to give him his opinion about his current condition. I worried about how the oncologist would be able to speak about the harsh reality of his physical condition yet maintain an element of hope of continued life for the immediate future which Eugene so desperately wanted, so that his optimism could be maintained. The doctor managed to do this and Eugene was satisfied with the information. He was now like a child, a feather in the breeze, as he tottered down the hospital corridor on the nurse's arm on his way to a pathology test.

On return home from the hospital, caring for him and providing the very best of comfort and nourishment became paramount. We resumed our routine, which included my reading from the Bible and from the daily prayer book which Helen, a friend, had given him and which were so comforting. He needed to be admitted to hospital again for a few days a few weeks later for more blood, and again we had to fight the hospital system to obtain a bed for him. The morphine was now making him confused and distracted in his weakened state.

Back home again, he was only able to take half of the communion host with wine. He now needed to be shaved and had had his last shower during the previous fortnight. He could only tolerate minimal liquid nourishment.

Each night before sleep for some weeks now, I would ask Eugene how the day had been for him. Generally, he replied that it had been good. However, one day, he had said it had been OK but he did not like the nurse sponging him down when I was out on a message. On arriving home that day, I had found him quite ruffled. Subsequently, he never let the nurses do this for him. He always said it was OK, as I did it for him.

On the day Eugene died, the GP was to have visited but decided to delay until the next day. Eugene had been in bed all day, which was the first day he had not sat in his chair in the bedroom. His body was twitching and he was unable to hold a glass. Helen visited in the early evening and cried when she saw his weakened and depleted state. She talked with Eugene about our twenty-five years of friendship. After her visit, he was terribly concerned that he had made her cry and could not bear that she was so upset on his behalf. She had cried because she loved him.

During Helen's visit, Eugene had started to become unwell and, soon after, it was obvious that a doctor should be called immediately. The doctor could not come immediately. However, the palliative nurse arrived and made Eugene as comfortable as she could. When the doctor arrived, he requested that the ambulance service provide oxygen. Eugene was most uncomfortable by now, as he was unable to breathe properly.

The peace of the past months was converted into an urgent flurry of activity – nurse sponging and rearranging the bed; doctor administering an enema and obtaining information about Eugene's immediate condition as he was an after-hours call-out doctor and had not visited previously; paramedics providing oxygen and deciding how to stretcher him through the narrow corridors of the house to the ambulance. They were all providing the best help but not necessarily meeting Eugene's needs, in that no one realised that he was dying.

During this time of making decisions and packing a hospital bag for him, his difficulty in breathing was intense. His large eyes met mine and I told him to breathe from the stomach as we had been taught in meditation. As the paramedics transferred him to the stretcher, I observed his physical appearance seemingly for the first time and I was amazed to see his condition. He was so thin and bony, with huge eyes, bloated stomach and legs. I had only seen his inner glow in the previous weeks and days as I had massaged his bony back and withered arms.

The paramedics told us that he was dying and I saw the life ebbing out of him just after we had exchanged glances, as he was fighting to breathe within the activity of moving him. We took him out to the ambulance and it was there that the doctor confirmed that Eugene had died. We brought him back to the bed, as I could not bear to have him in a strange place at this time. I assisted the palliative nurse in settling him in the bed. She asked that he be covered with something in a blue colour so that he would look his best.

The palliative care nurse was a wonderful comfort at this time. She interpreted Eugene's dream to mean that he was being told that he had almost finished the lessons of his journey that was just about complete.

When I observed that life had left Eugene as we were transferring him to the stretcher in the bedroom, my immediate reactions were of happiness that my poor boy need not suffer further. I thanked God for taking him before his condition became totally unbearable. His inner glow and calmness had belied the suffering he had already borne with such grace. I had willed him to be strong and, in taking up the challenge, Eugene had surpassed all of my expectations.

Eugene's life and last journey took its own particular timeframe. He took me with him on this privileged journey and left a wonderful gift of how to live life. He became a teacher of love, spirituality and dignity. When he had learnt and taught all of these things to others, he was allowed to die.

Eugene learned to deal with his cancer and turned it into a blessing for himself and for those he took along on his journey. He profoundly touched his friends, who will enjoy richer lives for the experience. He taught all of us to be aware of the things in life which are unimportant, and the wonderful privilege of loving and of being with someone on such a journey.

He showed us what unconditional love is and that we should adopt the positives and dump the negatives in life. He is the bond which has brought the cocoon of friends closer for ever more in the richness of sharing this experience. Eugene taught us that we should be treating each other in this way all the time, during all our lives, in all of our activities and in our caring of each other.

Eugene was always afraid of contracting cancer and, in confronting his biggest fear, he was able to turn this into a growth and learning time and to experience a lifetime of richness in his last six months.

Cancer taught Eugene how to live – to be resurrected – to alter his personality so as to experience a gentler, softer way of living.

These words, from The Prophet, by Kahlil Gibran, were in Eugene's diary; they were given to him by Jen Luddington to help him in his great journey of self-knowledge. He was to follow them to the letter:

You would know the secret of death.
But how shall you find it unless you seek it in the heart of life?

The owl whose night-bound eyes are blind unto the day cannot unveil the mystery of life.

If you would indeed behold the spirit of death, open your heart wide unto the body of life.

For life and death are one, even as the river and sea are one.

In the depth of your hopes and desires lies your silent knowledge of the beyond;

And life seeds dreaming beneath the snow your heart dreams of spring.

Trust the dreams, for in them is hidden the gate to eternity.

Your fear of death is but the trembling of the shepherd when he stands before the king whose hand is to be laid upon him in honour.

Is the shepherd not joyful beneath his trembling that he shall wear the mark of the king?

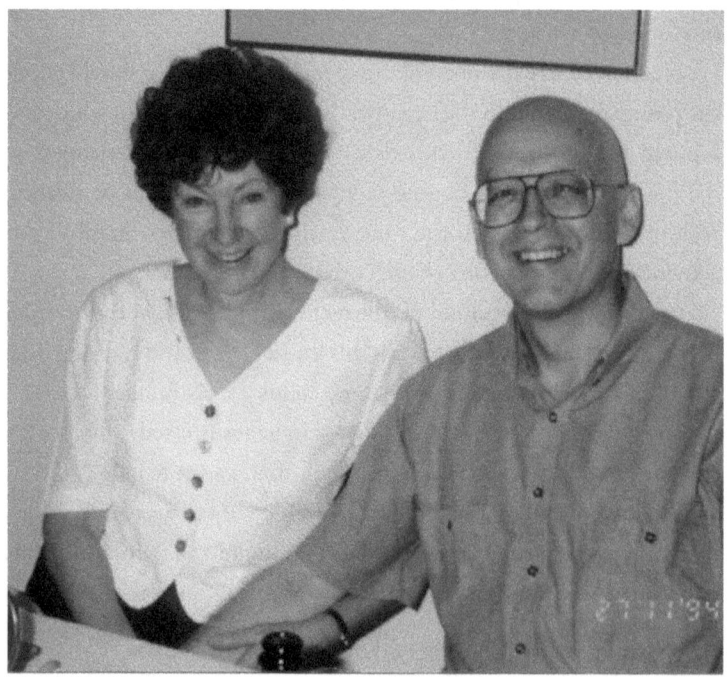

Nerelle and Eugene, November 1994

Yet is he not more mindful of his trembling?

For what is it to die but to stand naked in the wind and to melt into the sun?

And what is it to cease breathing but to free the breath from its restless tides, that it may rise and expand and seek God unencumbered?

Only when you drink from the river of silence shall you indeed sing.

And when you have reached the mountain top, then you shall begin to climb.

And when the earth shall claim your limbs, then shall you truly dance.

My Dear Bear

I spoke to you when I came into the bedroom the next morning after you had gone. You had not changed in looks from the previous night when the palliative care nurse and I had settled you to rest on the bed. However, I knew that your wonderful spirit had already gone. I think this occurred at about eleven-forty the previous night after we had settled your lifeless body.

I talked to you that next morning as I tidied up the ensuite from the previous night's chaos. I apologised for the never-ending noise of the washing machine which had so disturbed you in your illness. I had it running again this particular morning to clean the soiled towels. I showered in the ensuite and spoke to you while I dressed in the bedroom.

We had been through so much in the twenty years of marriage. As Gerry would explain it, the majority of the time were death years for you, and the last six months were wonderful days and months in which you had experienced your resurrection.

Like all of us, you were so bound up in the life role you had set for yourself so that you could get through your life's journey within your own comfort zone. Your love of the challenge of collecting books, reading them in the study, keeping your statistics on Australian Rules football, cricket and politics; enjoying the garden, favourite places in Canberra, the movies, the plays, the restaurants, the holidays and the visits to the Blue Mountains, Sydney, Melbourne and Perth were your buffers against your uncertain feelings about your career in the Public Service.

In later years, the stresses of work and your inability to move out of your comfort zone meant that your life was out of balance in that you felt you were losing your humour. Your self-esteem was low and you were stressed, impatient, negative and unhappy. I felt that you would never be able to change this situation for yourself.

We planned your journey through cancer together and completed the journey with top marks. You underwent a major change in doing for yourself what you had never been able to achieve before. You found out how to love yourself and in doing that you grew to be able to feel and to show your love for your friends. You experienced feelings. Even in the midst of your fear of being the centre of attention you thanked the parishioners of the Healing Ministry for their generosity. You grew to accept their generosity and it came naturally to you to give them and God thanks from your heart. You learned these lessons, which resulted in feeling love and experiencing growth.

Tom, your nephew, taught you the lesson of patience and what is important in life during his visit in your last months. You never did have much patience with timeframes or deadlines, and you intensely worried about missing a train or being able to carry out a task around the house without angst. Your love for Tom allowed you to make the decision to come to terms with the difference between yourself and an exuberant eight-year-old boy in order to enjoy his presence. You built on the knowledge you gained from Gerry Manion and Jen Luddington in allowing Tom the freedom to be himself whilst you minimised your stress and impatience with him.

In contrast to earlier years, you also learned to be patient with me when I cared for you during your illness. George forever wanted to make your life more comfortable in installing phones, bringing comfortable chairs, helping with an air conditioner and giving you a buzzer to call me from another room. When George wanted to install in the bedroom the buzzer by which you could summon me, you said you did not want to do this to me as I had so much to do in caring for you. You were also worried about the difficulty you thought I must surely be experiencing in providing you with adequate and nutritious food when your ability to take food was minimal. In effect, I was experiencing my higher being in the love I felt when I was preparing your food. Nothing was a problem for me – I had so much strength of mind and body for you. In turn, you were able to employ a gentler, softer way in interacting with me. This was so out of character with your usual impatient self. The growth in you was a delight to watch. You became so soft and gentle and your smile was full of meaning. You found your purpose and meaning in life.

I so enjoyed planning your health strategy with you and boosting your positiveness because you became so receptive to being positive. You were so positive you almost wore yourself out by not letting go at the end of your time.

I thank God for the heart attack which occurred when it did, as your last day was drained of energy. God looked after you in your timing to die. You were so close to him. I can see your face when you said, 'Please, please, please,' for him to ease the pain and 'Thank you, thank you, thank you,' when it eased. Your prayers from your spirit were an inspiration to everyone, even your minister, and you were an inspiration to your friends in the Cancer Support Group at the Cancer Society when they saw how you dealt with your cancer care with such grace. They described you as being very noble.

You were zinging along with God, enjoying hearing the

words of the Bible and Helen's daily prayer book through my reading or from a tape. This is all you wanted in your last days. You were so close to God.

I think he was telling you in that dream that you were well because you had completed your spiritual journey and had been made well and would experience happiness and love soon with him. I have learned in sharing your last months with you that the Higher Self wherein we are granted honour and nobility is paramount. Gerry's lessons were about all of this.

In your illness you were stripped down to your essential lovely self. You had such grace and dignity in your pain that I could not see your deterioration and told people you were feeling much the same. You would say, 'Tell it like it is — I am worse'! Maybe it was hope that would not let me face your deterioration. You worried that friends would expect you to be in better health than you were. When your work colleagues visited in the last weeks, you worried that you could not get up from the chair and be dressed in your day clothes. In previous times, you worried about the small things such as a cut or an ache. You bore the big thing with grace. I remember how your body looked and how the doctor described your depleted state the night you died. Only then did I comprehend fully how your body had deteriorated and had become so misshapen through the tumour and fluid in your legs. Only then when your spirit had left your body did I see your depleted state. With you in there, your will and positiveness and wonderful spirit masked all the physical changes for me. I only saw your real self shining through, the real self who kissed my lips and hands so strongly in such a weakened physical state and told me you loved me in every way.

You showed such emotion when I told you it was a privilege to spend this time together and there would never be another time so wonderful and uplifting. You were so pleased I gave you the variety of Christmas presents chosen with so much love. I had chosen special items which represented that you still had a future, such as the wristwatch, the diaries to record each day, the one minute meditation book and the cheerful caps to wear whilst your hair was growing back. You so enjoyed the flowers which I gave you. It was so wonderful to find all these natural responses in you which, outside of your resurrection time, you could not have shown. You were a joy to be with.

I must keep the purity of this time we had together in my heart for the rest of my life. You taught me what lightness of being means. It means that I must remember not to 'sweat the small stuff' and recognise it's all small stuff. I must also continue to stay within a supportive environment and dump the negative and non-supportive environment and listen to the spirituality of my higher self.

The greatest emotion we had for us during the six months of our journey together, my Dear Bear, was unconditional love. Our love for each other was strengthened by many years of being together, by being in your words 'soulmates' and instinctively knowing what was in each heart. This togetherness all came together so perfectly in your resurrection. The love of friends was also wonderful, as was the love they felt for each other in the experience. They made a cocoon of love around us and you responded wonderfully to it. I also learned to trust friends and receive their love with an open heart.

I was go glad God took you with mercy. I hope you were ready. I think you were still holding on, as life is wonderful. I think that you were more than prepared, however, and know that you accepted wholeheartedly God's loving place. You had a vision of my attaining my PhD even before that thought entered into my head. You could already visualise my achieving this before it entered into my consciousness. You were so supportive of my studies from the time we studied Russian together in 1972 and I went on to complete my undergraduate studies. You showed me how organised you were in your approach to studies. You were a good teacher and took such delight in discussing all the pieces of information you retained from being an avid reader while at the same time castigating yourself for not reading enough and not retaining the information to the extent you wanted. You were very proud of my achievements. You wanted to buy more flowers for me. You were so appreciative of my caring for you. Oh, to be able to see your calm and wonderful smile. Bear, how I love and miss you. I feel that you will watch over me and care for me for the rest of my life.

Never let me forget how it was, and the lessons you taught me on your wonderful journey of resurrection. I can also remember the elation I felt the day after you died and my feeling of: WE DID IT – WE COULD NOT HAVE DONE IT BETTER. You left me a wonderful gift. Please let this feeling stay with me forever.

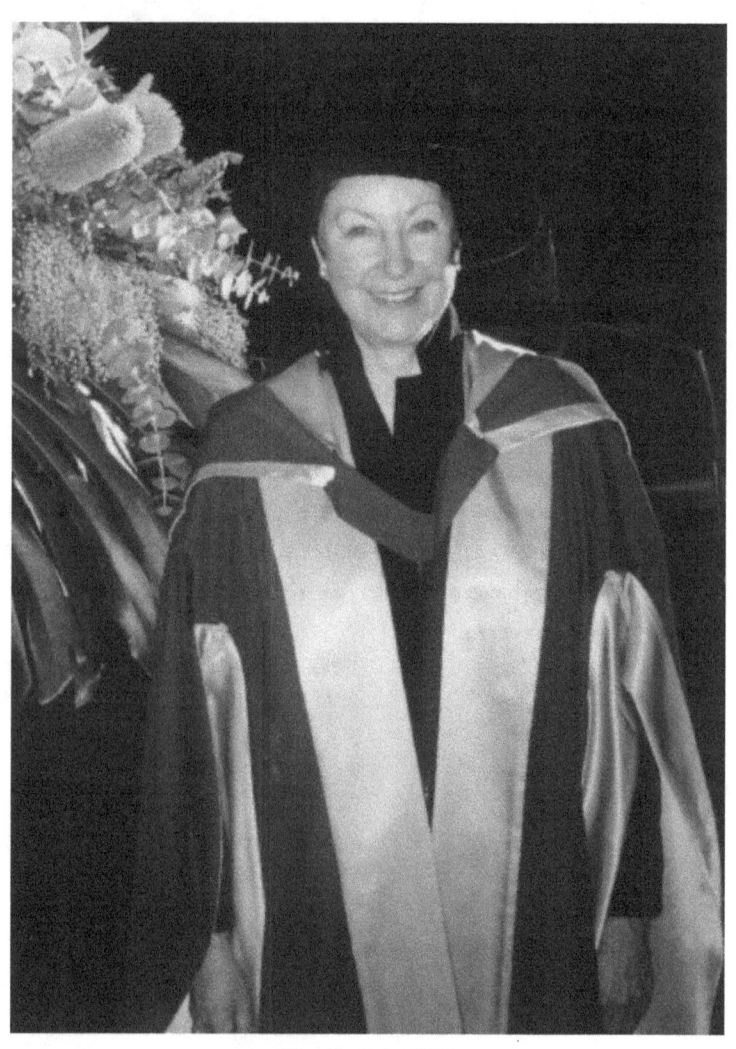

Nerelle, July 2001

Bibliography

Bryant, B. 1990. *Cancer and Consciousness.* Sligo Press, Boston.

Ram Dass. *Journey of Awakening. A Meditator's Guidebook.*

Gawler, I. 1984. *You Can Conquer Cancer. Prevention and Management.* Hill of Content, Melbourne.

Glennon, J. 1993. *How Can I Find Healing?* Hodder & Stoughton, Sydney.

Jeffers, S. 1993. *Feel the Fear and Do It Anyway.* Arrow, London.

Kuhlman, K. *I Believe in Miracles. God's Power to Heal Today.*

Manion, G. 1994. *Cancer Care Programme.* Sydney.

Simonton, O. Carl, Henson, R., and Hampton, B. 1992. *The Healing Journey. Restoring Health and Harmony to Body, Mind, and Spirit.* Bantam Books, New York.

Acknowledgements

Gerard Manion for the Preface
Dr Glen Lewis for back cover notes
George Fava for photographs
ACT Writers Centre for advice
Stephen Matthews for publishing support

www.ingramcontent.com/pod-product-compliance
Lightning Source LLC
Chambersburg PA
CBHW071126030426
42336CB00013BA/2222